MW00509451

INDIAN RECIPES 2021

TASTY RECIPES OF THE INDIAN TRADITION

MELANIA WHITE

Table of Contents

Tandoori Potato 12

    Ingredients 12

    Method 12

Corn Curry 14

    Ingredients 14

    Method 15

Masala Green Pepper 16

    Ingredients 16

    Method 17

No-oil Bottle Gourd 18

    Ingredients 18

    Method 18

Okra with Yoghurt 19

    Ingredients 19

    Method 20

Sautéed Karela 21

    Ingredients 21

    Method 22

Cabbage with Peas 23

    Ingredients 23

    Method 23

Potatoes in Tomato Sauce 24

    Ingredients 24

Method.. 24

Matar Palak 25

Ingredients 25

Method.. 26

Masala Cabbage 27

Ingredients 27

Method.. 28

Dry Spicy Cauliflower 29

Ingredients 29

Method.. 30

Mushroom Curry... 31

Ingredients 31

Method.. 32

Baingan Bharta.. 33

Ingredients 33

Method.. 34

Vegetable Hyderabadi... 35

Ingredients 35

For the spice mixture: 35

Method.. 36

Kaddu Bhaji* 37

Ingredients 37

Method.. 38

Muthia nu Shak 39

Ingredients 39

Method.. 40

Pumpkin Koot.. 41

Ingredients 41

Method 42

Rassa 43

Ingredients 43

Method 44

Doodhi Manpasand 45

Ingredients 45

Method 46

Tomato Chokha 47

Ingredients 47

Method 47

Baingan Chokha 48

Ingredients 48

Method 48

Cauliflower & Peas Curry 49

Ingredients 49

Method 49

Aloo Methi ki Sabzi 50

Ingredients 50

Method 50

Sweet & Sour Karela 51

Ingredients 51

Method 52

Karela Koshimbir 53

Ingredients 53

Method 53

Karela Curry 54

Ingredients 54

Method... 55

Chilli Cauliflower 56

Ingredients 56

Method... 56

Nutty Curry.. 57

Ingredients 57

Method... 58

Daikon Leaves Bhaaji.. 59

Ingredients 59

Method... 59

Chhole Aloo 60

Ingredients 60

Method... 61

Peanut Curry 62

Ingredients 62

Method... 63

French Beans Upkari 64

Ingredients 64

Method... 64

Karatey Ambadey.. 65

Ingredients 65

Method... 66

Kadhai Paneer 67

Ingredients 67

Method... 67

Kathirikkai Vangi 68

Ingredients 68

Method 69

Pitla 70

Ingredients 70

Method 71

Cauliflower Masala 72

Ingredients 72

For the sauce: 72

Method 73

Shukna Kacha Pepe 74

Ingredients 74

Method 75

Dry Okra 76

Ingredients 76

Method 76

Moghlai Cauliflower 77

Ingredients 77

Method 77

Bhapa Shorshe Baingan 78

Ingredients 78

Method 79

Baked Vegetables in Spicy Sauce 80

Ingredients 80

Method 81

Tasty Tofu 82

Ingredients 82

Method 82

Aloo Baingan 83

    Ingredients 83

    Method... 84

Sugar Snap Pea Curry 85

    Ingredients 85

    Method... 85

Potato Pumpkin Curry... 86

    Ingredients 86

    Method... 87

Egg Thoran 88

    Ingredients 88

    Method... 89

Baingan Lajawab 90

    Ingredients 90

    Method... 91

Veggie Bahar 92

    Ingredients 92

    Method... 93

Stuffed Vegetables... 94

    Ingredients 94

    For the filling: 94

    Method... 95

Singhi Aloo 96

    Ingredients 96

    Method... 96

Sindhi Curry.. 97

    Ingredients 97

Method 98

Dum Gobhi..99

Ingredients..99

Method 99

Chhole...100

Ingredients..100

Method 101

Aubergine Curry with Onion & Potato 102

Ingredients..102

Method 103

Simple Bottle Gourd 104

Ingredients..104

Method 104

Mixed Vegetable Curry...105

Ingredients..105

Method 106

Dry Mixed Vegetables...107

Ingredients..107

Method 108

Dry Potatoes & Peas 109

Ingredients..109

Method 109

Dhokar Dhalna...110

Ingredients..110

Method 111

Spicy Fried Potatoes 112

Ingredients..112

Method...112

Tandoori Potato

Serves 4

Ingredients

16 large potatoes, peeled

Refined vegetable oil to deep fry

3 tbsp finely chopped tomatoes

1 tbsp coriander leaves, chopped

1 tsp garam masala

100g/3½oz Cheddar cheese, grated

Salt to taste

Juice of 2 lemons

Method

- Scoop out the potatoes. Reserve the flesh and the hollowed parts.

- Heat the oil in a frying pan. Add the hollowed potatoes. Fry them on a medium heat till they turn golden brown. Set aside.

- To the same oil, add the scooped potatoes and all the remaining ingredients, except the lemon juice. Sauté on a low heat for 5 minutes.

- Stuff this mixture inside the hollow potatoes.

- Bake the stuffed potatoes in an oven at 200°C (400°F, Gas Mark 6) for 5 minutes.

- Sprinkle the lemon juice on top of the potatoes. Serve hot.

Corn Curry

Serves 4

Ingredients

1 large potato, boiled and mashed

500g/1lb 2oz tomato purée

3 tbsp refined vegetable oil

8 curry leaves

2 tbsp besan*

1 tsp ginger paste

½ tsp turmeric

Salt to taste

1 tsp garam masala

1 tsp chilli powder

3 tsp sugar

250ml/8fl oz water

4 corn on the cobs, chopped into 3 pieces each and boiled

Method

- Mix the potato mash thoroughly with the tomato purée. Set aside.

- Heat the oil in a saucepan. Add the curry leaves. Let them crackle for 10 seconds. Add the besan and ginger paste. Fry on a low heat till brown.

- Add the potato-tomato mixture and all the remaining ingredients except the corn. Simmer for 3-4 minutes.

- Add the corn pieces. Mix well. Simmer for 8-10 minutes. Serve hot.

Masala Green Pepper

Serves 4

Ingredients

1½ tbsp refined vegetable oil

1 tsp garam masala

¼ tsp turmeric

½ tsp ginger paste

½ tsp garlic paste

1 large onion, finely chopped

1 tomato, finely chopped

4 large green peppers, julienned

125g/4½oz yoghurt

Salt to taste

Method

- Heat the oil in a saucepan. Add the garam masala, turmeric, ginger paste and garlic paste. Fry this mixture on a medium heat for 2 minutes.

- Add the onion. Fry till it is translucent.

- Add the tomato and green peppers. Fry for 2-3 minutes. Add the yoghurt and salt. Mix well. Cook for 6-7 minutes. Serve hot.

No-oil Bottle Gourd

Serves 4

Ingredients

500g/1lb 2oz bottle gourd*, skinned and chopped

2 tomatoes, finely chopped

1 large onion, finely chopped

1 tsp ginger paste

1 tsp garlic paste

2 green chillies, finely chopped

½ tsp ground coriander

½ tsp ground cumin

25g/scant 1oz coriander leaves, finely chopped

120ml/4fl oz water

Salt to taste

Method

- Mix all the ingredients together. Cook in a saucepan on a low heat for 20 minutes. Serve hot.

Okra with Yoghurt

Serves 4

Ingredients

3 tbsp refined vegetable oil

½ tsp cumin seeds

500g/1lb 2oz okra, chopped

½ tsp chilli powder

¼ tsp turmeric

2 green chillies, slit lengthways

1 tsp ginger, julienned

200g/7oz yoghurt

1 tsp besan*, dissolved in 1 tbsp water

Salt to taste

1 tbsp coriander leaves, finely chopped

Method

- Heat the oil in a saucepan. Add the cumin seeds. Let them splutter for 15 seconds.

- Add the okra, chilli powder, turmeric, green chillies and ginger.

- Cook on a low heat for 20 minutes, stirring occasionally.

- Add the yoghurt, besan mixture and salt. Cook for 5 minutes.

- Garnish the okra with the coriander leaves. Serve hot.

Sautéed Karela

(Sautéed Bitter Gourd)

Serves 4

Ingredients

4 medium-sized bitter gourds*

Salt to taste

1½ tbsp refined vegetable oil

½ tsp mustard seeds

½ tsp turmeric

½ tsp ginger paste

½ tsp garlic paste

2 large onions, finely chopped

½ tsp chilli powder

¾ tsp jaggery*, grated

Method

- Peel the bitter gourds and slit into halves, lengthways. Discard the seeds and thinly slice each half. Add the salt and set aside for 20 minutes. Squeeze out the water. Set aside again.

- Heat the oil in a saucepan. Add the mustard seeds. Let them splutter for 15 seconds.

- Add the remaining ingredients and fry them on a medium heat for 2-3 minutes. Add the bitter gourd. Mix well. Cook for 5 minutes on a low heat. Serve hot.

Cabbage with Peas

Serves 4

Ingredients

1 tbsp refined vegetable oil

1 tsp mustard seeds

2 green chillies, slit lengthways

¼ tsp turmeric

400g/14oz cabbage, finely shredded

125g/4½oz fresh peas

Salt to taste

2 tbsp desiccated coconut

Method

- Heat the oil in a saucepan. Add the mustard seeds and green chillies. Let them splutter for 15 seconds.
- Add the remaining ingredients, except the coconut. Cook on a low heat for 10 minutes.
- Add the coconut. Mix well. Serve hot.

Potatoes in Tomato Sauce

Serves 4

Ingredients

2 tbsp refined vegetable oil

1 tsp cumin seeds

Pinch of asafoetida

½ tsp turmeric

4 large potatoes, boiled and diced

4 tomatoes, finely chopped

1 tsp chilli powder

Salt to taste

1 tbsp coriander leaves, chopped

Method

- Heat the oil in a saucepan. Add the cumin seeds, asafoetida and turmeric. Let them splutter for 15 seconds.
- Add the remaining ingredients, except the coriander leaves. Mix well. Cook on a low heat for 10 minutes. Garnish with the coriander leaves. Serve hot.

Matar Palak

(Peas and Spinach)

Serves 4

Ingredients

400g/14oz spinach, steamed and chopped

2 green chillies

4-5 tbsp refined vegetable oil

1 tsp cumin seeds

1 pinch of asafoetida

1 tsp turmeric

1 large onion, finely chopped

1 tomato, finely chopped

1 large potato, diced

Salt to taste

200g/7oz green peas

Method

- Grind together the spinach and chillies to a fine paste. Set aside.

- Heat the oil in a saucepan. Add the cumin seeds, asafoetida and turmeric. Let them splutter for 15 seconds.

- Add the onion. Fry on a medium heat till it turns translucent.

- Add the remaining ingredients. Mix well. Cook on a low heat for 7-8 minutes, stirring occasionally.

- Add the spinach paste. Simmer for 5 minutes. Serve hot.

Masala Cabbage

(Spicy Cabbage)

Serves 4

Ingredients

3 tbsp refined vegetable oil

1 tsp cumin seeds

¼ tsp turmeric

1 tsp garlic paste

1 tsp ginger paste

1 large onion, finely chopped

1 tomato, finely chopped

½ tsp chilli powder

Salt to taste

400g/14oz cabbage, finely chopped

Method

- Heat the oil in a saucepan. Add the cumin seeds and turmeric. Let them splutter for 15 seconds. Add the garlic paste, ginger paste and onion. Fry on a medium heat for 2-3 minutes.

- Add the tomato, chilli powder, salt and cabbage. Mix well. Cover with a lid and cook on a low heat for 10-15 minutes. Serve hot.

Dry Spicy Cauliflower

Serves 4

Ingredients

750g/1lb 10oz cauliflower florets

Salt to taste

Pinch of turmeric

4 bay leaves

750ml/1¼ pints water

2 tbsp refined vegetable oil

4 cloves

4 green cardamom pods

1 large onion, sliced

1 tsp ginger paste

1 tsp garlic paste

1 tsp garam masala

½ tsp chilli powder

¼ tsp ground black pepper

10 cashew nuts, ground

2 tbsp yoghurt

3 tbsp tomato purée

3 tbsp butter

60ml/2fl oz single cream

Method

- Cook the cauliflower with the salt, turmeric, bay leaves and water in a saucepan on a medium heat for 10 minutes. Drain and arrange the florets in an ovenproof dish. Set aside.

- Heat the oil in a saucepan. Add the cloves and cardamom. Let them splutter for 15 seconds.

- Add the onion, ginger paste and garlic paste. Fry for a minute.

- Add the garam masala, chilli powder, pepper and cashew nuts. Fry for 1-2 minutes.

- Add the yoghurt and tomato purée. Mix thoroughly. Add the butter and cream. Stir for a minute. Remove from the heat.

- Pour this over the cauliflower florets. Bake at 150°C (300°F, Gas Mark 2) in a pre-heated oven for 8-10 minutes. Serve hot.

Mushroom Curry

Serves 4

Ingredients

3 tbsp refined vegetable oil

2 large onions, grated

1 tsp ginger paste

1 tsp garlic paste

½ tsp turmeric

1 tsp chilli powder

1 tsp ground coriander

400g/14oz mushrooms, quartered

200g/7oz peas

2 tomatoes, finely chopped

½ tsp garam masala

Salt to taste

20 cashew nuts, ground

240ml/6fl oz water

Method

- Heat the oil in a saucepan. Add the onions. Fry them till they are brown.

- Add the ginger paste, garlic paste, turmeric, chilli powder and ground coriander. Sauté on a medium heat for a minute.

- Add the remaining ingredients. Mix well. Cover with a lid and simmer for 8-10 minutes. Serve hot.

Baingan Bharta

(Roasted Aubergine)

Serves 4

Ingredients

1 large aubergine

3 tbsp refined vegetable oil

1 large onion, finely chopped

3 green chillies, slit lengthways

¼ tsp turmeric

Salt to taste

½ tsp garam masala

1 tomato, finely chopped

Method

- Pierce the aubergine all over with a fork and grill it for 25 minutes. Once it has cooled, discard the roasted skin and mash the flesh. Set aside.

- Heat the oil in a saucepan. Add the onion and green chillies. Fry on a medium heat for 2 minutes.

- Add the turmeric, salt, garam masala and tomato. Mix well. Fry for 5 minutes. Add the mashed aubergine. Mix well.

- Cook on a low heat for 8 minutes, stirring occasionally. Serve hot.

Vegetable Hyderabadi

Serves 4

Ingredients

2 tbsp refined vegetable oil

½ tsp mustard seeds

1 large onion, finely chopped

400g/14oz frozen, mixed vegetables

½ tsp turmeric

Salt to taste

For the spice mixture:

2.5cm/1in root ginger

8 garlic cloves

2 cloves

2.5cm/1in cinnamon

1 tsp fenugreek seeds

3 green chillies

4 tbsp fresh coconut, grated

10 cashew nuts

Method

- Grind all the ingredients of the spice mixture together. Set aside.

- Heat the oil in a saucepan. Add the mustard seeds. Let them splutter for 15 seconds. Add the onion and fry till brown.

- Add the remaining ingredients and the ground spice mixture. Mix well. Cook on a low heat for 8-10 minutes. Serve hot.

Kaddu Bhaji*

(Dry Red Pumpkin)

Serves 4

Ingredients

3 tbsp refined vegetable oil

½ tsp cumin seeds

¼ tsp fenugreek seeds

600g/1lb 5oz pumpkin, thinly sliced

Salt to taste

½ tsp roasted ground cumin

½ tsp chilli powder

¼ tsp turmeric

1 tsp amchoor*

1 tsp sugar

Method

- Heat the oil in a saucepan. Add the cumin and fenugreek seeds. Let them splutter for 15 seconds. Add the pumpkin and salt. Mix well. Cover with a lid and cook on a medium heat for 8 minutes.

- Uncover and lightly crush with the back of a spoon. Add the remaining ingredients. Mix well. Cook for 5 minutes. Serve hot.

Muthia nu Shak

(Fenugreek Dumplings in Sauce)

Serves 4

Ingredients

200g/7oz fresh fenugreek leaves, finely chopped

Salt to taste

125g/4½oz wholemeal flour

125g/4½oz besan*

2 green chillies, finely chopped

1 tsp ginger paste

3 tsp sugar

Juice of 1 lemon

½ tsp garam masala

½ tsp turmeric

Pinch of bicarbonate of soda

3 tbsp refined vegetable oil

½ tsp ajowan seeds

½ tsp mustard seeds

Pinch of asafoetida

250ml/8fl oz water

Method

- Mix the fenugreek leaves with the salt. Set aside for 10 minutes. Squeeze out the moisture.

- Mix the fenugreek leaves with the flour, besan, green chillies, ginger paste, sugar, lemon juice, garam masala, turmeric and bicarbonate of soda. Knead into a soft dough.

- Divide the dough into 30 walnut-sized balls. Flatten slightly to form the muthias. Set aside.

- Heat the oil in a saucepan. Add the ajowan seeds, mustard seeds and asafoetida. Let them splutter for 15 seconds.

- Add the muthias and water.

- Cover with a lid and simmer for 10-15 minutes. Serve hot.

Pumpkin Koot

(Pumpkin in Lentil Curry)

Serves 4

Ingredients

50g/1¾oz fresh coconut, grated

1 tsp cumin seeds

2 red chillies

150g/5½oz mung dhal*, soaked for 30 minutes and drained

2 tbsp chana dhal*

Salt to taste

500ml/16fl oz water

2 tbsp refined vegetable oil

250g/9oz pumpkin, diced

¼ tsp turmeric

Method

- Grind the coconut, cumin seeds and red chillies to a paste. Set aside.

- Mix the dhals with the salt and water. Cook this mixture in a saucepan on a medium heat for 40 minutes. Set aside.

- Heat the oil in a saucepan. Add the pumpkin, turmeric, boiled dhals and the coconut paste. Mix well. Simmer for 10 minutes. Serve hot.

Rassa

(Cauliflower and Peas in Sauce)

Serves 4

Ingredients

2 tbsp refined vegetable oil plus extra for deep frying

250g/9oz cauliflower florets

2 tbsp fresh coconut, grated

1cm/½in root ginger, crushed

4-5 green chillies, slit lengthways

2-3 tomatoes, finely chopped

400g/14oz frozen peas

1 tsp sugar

Salt to taste

Method

- Heat the oil for deep frying in a saucepan. Add the cauliflower. Deep fry on a medium heat till golden brown. Drain and set aside.

- Grind the coconut, ginger, green chillies and tomatoes. Heat 2 tbsp oil in a saucepan. Add this paste and fry for 1-2 minutes.

- Add the cauliflower and the remaining ingredients. Mix well. Cook on a low heat for 4-5 minutes. Serve hot.

Doodhi Manpasand

(Bottle Gourd in Sauce)

Serves 4

Ingredients

3 tbsp refined vegetable oil

3 dried red chillies

1 large onion, finely chopped

500g/1lb 2oz bottle gourd*, chopped

¼ tsp turmeric

2 tsp ground coriander

1 tsp ground cumin

½ tsp chilli powder

½ tsp garam masala

2.5cm/1in root ginger, finely chopped

2 tomatoes, finely chopped

1 green pepper, cored, deseeded and finely chopped

Salt to taste

2 tsp coriander leaves, finely chopped

Method

- Heat the oil in a saucepan. Fry the red chillies and onion for 2 minutes.
- Add the remaining ingredients, except the coriander leaves. Mix well. Cook on a low heat for 5-7 minutes. Garnish with the coriander leaves. Serve hot.

Tomato Chokha

(Tomato Compote)

Serves 4

Ingredients

6 large tomatoes

2 tbsp refined vegetable oil

1 big onion, finely chopped

8 garlic cloves, finely chopped

1 green chilli, finely chopped

½ tsp chilli powder

10g/¼oz coriander leaves, finely chopped

Salt to taste

Method

- Grill the tomatoes for 10 minutes. Peel and crush to a pulp. Set aside.
- Heat the oil in a saucepan. Add the onion, garlic and green chilli. Fry for 2-3 minutes. Add the remaining ingredients and the tomato pulp. Mix well. Cover with a lid and cook for 5-6 minutes. Serve hot.

Baingan Chokha

(Aubergine Compote)

Serves 4

Ingredients

1 large aubergine

2 tbsp refined vegetable oil

1 small onion, chopped

8 garlic cloves, finely chopped

1 green chilli, finely chopped

1 tomato, finely chopped

60g/2oz corn kernels, boiled

10g/¼oz coriander leaves, finely chopped

Salt to taste

Method

- Pierce the aubergine all over with a fork. Grill for 10-15 minutes. Peel and crush to a pulp. Set aside.
- Heat the oil in a saucepan. Add the onion, garlic and green chilli. Fry them on a medium heat for 5 minutes.
- Add the remaining ingredients and the aubergine pulp. Mix well. Cook for 3-4 minutes. Serve hot.

Cauliflower & Peas Curry

Serves 4

Ingredients

3 tbsp refined vegetable oil

¼ tsp turmeric

3 green chillies, slit lengthways

1 tsp ground coriander

2.5cm/1in root ginger, grated

250g/9oz cauliflower florets

400g/14oz fresh green peas

60ml/2fl oz water

Salt to taste

1 tbsp coriander leaves, finely chopped

Method

- Heat the oil in a saucepan. Add the turmeric, green chillies, ground coriander and ginger. Fry on a medium heat for a minute.
- Add the remaining ingredients, except the coriander leaves. Mix well Simmer for 10 minutes.
- Garnish with the coriander leaves. Serve hot.

Aloo Methi ki Sabzi

(Potato and Fenugreek Curry)

Serves 4

Ingredients

100g/3½oz fenugreek leaves, chopped

Salt to taste

4 tbsp refined vegetable oil

1 tsp cumin seeds

5-6 green chillies

¼ tsp turmeric

Pinch of asafoetida

6 large potatoes, boiled and chopped

Method

- Mix the fenugreek leaves with the salt. Set aside for 10 minutes.
- Heat the oil in a saucepan. Add the cumin seeds, chillies and turmeric. Let them splutter for 15 seconds.
- Add the remaining ingredients and the fenugreek leaves. Mix well. Cook for 8-10 minutes on a low heat. Serve hot.

Sweet & Sour Karela

Serves 4

Ingredients

500g/1lb 2oz bitter gourds*

Salt to taste

750ml/1¼ pints water

1cm/½in root ginger

10 garlic cloves

4 large onions, chopped

4 tbsp refined vegetable oil

Pinch of asafoetida

½ tsp turmeric

1 tsp ground coriander

1 tsp ground cumin

1 tsp tamarind paste

2 tbsp jaggery*, grated

Method

- Peel the bitter gourds. Slice and soak them in salty water for 1 hour. Rinse and squeeze out the excess water. Wash and set aside.

- Grind the ginger, garlic and onions to a paste. Set aside.

- Heat the oil in a saucepan. Add the asafoetida. Let it splutter for 15 seconds. Add the ginger-onion paste and the remaining ingredients. Mix well. Fry for 3-4 minutes. Add the bitter gourds. Mix well. Cover with a lid and cook on a low heat for 8-10 minutes. Serve hot.

Karela Koshimbir

(Crispy Crushed Bitter Gourd)

Serves 4

Ingredients

500g/1lb 2oz bitter gourds*, peeled

Salt to taste

Refined vegetable oil for frying

2 medium-sized onions, chopped

50g/1¾oz coriander leaves, chopped

3 green chillies, finely chopped

½ fresh coconut, grated

1 tbsp lemon juice

Method

- Slice the bitter gourds. Rub the salt on them and set aside for 2-3 hours.
- Heat the oil in a saucepan. Add the bitter gourds and fry on a medium heat till brown and crispy. Drain, cool a little and crush with your fingers.
- Mix the remaining ingredients in a bowl. Add the gourds and serve while they are still warm.

Karela Curry

(Bitter Gourd Curry)

Serves 4

Ingredients

½ coconut

2 red chillies

1 tsp cumin seeds

3 tbsp refined vegetable oil

1 pinch of asafoetida

2 large onions, finely chopped

2 green chillies, finely chopped

Salt to taste

½ tsp turmeric

500g/1lb 2oz bitter gourds*, peeled and chopped

2 tomatoes, finely chopped

Method

- Grate half of the coconut and chop the rest. Set aside.
- Dry roast (see cooking techniques) the grated coconut, red chillies and cumin seeds. Cool and grind together to a fine paste. Set aside.
- Heat the oil in a frying pan. Add the asafoetida, onions, green chillies, salt, turmeric and chopped coconut. Fry for 3 minutes, stirring frequently.
- Add the bitter gourds and tomatoes. Cook for 3-4 minutes.
- Add the ground coconut paste. Cook for 5-7 minutes and serve hot.

Chilli Cauliflower

Serves 4

Ingredients

3 tbsp refined vegetable oil

5cm/2in root ginger, finely chopped

12 garlic cloves, finely chopped

1 cauliflower, chopped into florets

5 red chillies, quartered and deseeded

6 spring onions, halved

3 tomatoes, blanched and chopped

Salt to taste

Method

- Heat the oil in a saucepan. Add the ginger and garlic. Fry on a medium heat for a minute.
- Add the cauliflower and red chillies. Stir-fry for 5 minutes.
- Add the remaining ingredients. Mix well. Cook on a low heat for 7-8 minutes. Serve hot.

Nutty Curry

Serves 4

Ingredients

4 tbsp ghee

10g/¼oz cashew nuts

10g/¼oz almonds, blanched

10-12 peanuts

5-6 raisins

10 pistachios

10 walnuts, chopped

2.5cm/1in root ginger, grated

6 garlic cloves, crushed

4 small onions, finely chopped

4 tomatoes, finely chopped

4 dates, de-seeded and sliced

½ tsp turmeric

125g/4½oz khoya*

1 tsp garam masala

Salt to taste

75g/2½ Cheddar cheese, grated

1 tbsp coriander leaves, chopped

Method

- Heat the ghee in a frying pan. Add all the nuts and fry them on a medium heat till they turn golden brown. Drain and set aside.

- In the same ghee, fry the ginger, garlic and onion till brown.

- Add the fried nuts and all the remaining ingredients, except the cheese and coriander leaves. Cover with a lid. Cook on a low heat for 5 minutes.

- Garnish with the cheese and coriander leaves. Serve hot.

Daikon Leaves Bhaaji

Serves 4

Ingredients

2 tbsp refined vegetable oil

¼ tsp ground cumin

2 red chillies, broken into bits

Pinch of asafoetida

400g/14oz daikon leaves*, chopped

300g/10oz chana dhal*, soaked for 1 hour

1 tsp jaggery*, grated

¼ tsp turmeric

Salt to taste

Method

- Heat the oil in a saucepan. Add the cumin, red chillies and asafoetida.
- Let them splutter for 15 seconds. Add the remaining ingredients. Mix well. Cook on a low heat for 10-15 minutes. Serve hot.

Chhole Aloo

(Chickpea and Potato Curry)

Serves 4

Ingredients

500g/1lb 2oz chickpeas, soaked overnight

Pinch of bicarbonate of soda

Salt to taste

1 litre/1¾ pints water

3 tbsp ghee

2.5cm/1in root ginger, julienned

2 large onions, grated, plus 1 small onion, sliced

2 tomatoes, diced

1 tsp garam masala

1 tsp ground cumin, dry roasted (see cooking techniques)

½ tsp ground green cardamom

½ tsp turmeric

2 large potatoes, boiled and diced

2 tsp tamarind paste

1 tbsp coriander leaves, chopped

Method

- Cook the chickpeas with the bicarbonate of soda, salt and water in a saucepan on a medium heat for 45 minutes. Drain and set aside.
- Heat the ghee in a saucepan. Add the ginger and grated onions. Fry till translucent. Add the remaining ingredients, except the coriander leaves and sliced onion. Mix well. Add the chickpeas and cook for 7-8 minutes.
- Garnish with the coriander leaves and sliced onion. Serve hot.

Peanut Curry

Serves 4

Ingredients

1 tsp poppy seeds

1 tsp coriander seeds

1 tsp cumin seeds

2 red chillies

25g/scant 1oz fresh coconut, grated

3 tbsp ghee

2 small onions, grated

900g/2lb peanuts, pounded

1 tsp amchoor*

½ tsp turmeric

1 big tomato, blanched and chopped

2 tsp jaggery*, grated

500ml/16fl oz water

Salt to taste

15g/½oz coriander leaves, chopped

Method

- Grind the poppy seeds, coriander seeds, cumin seeds, red chillies and coconut to a fine paste. Set aside.
- Heat the ghee in a saucepan. Add the onions. Fry till translucent.
- Add the ground paste and the remaining ingredients, except the coriander leaves. Mix well. Simmer for 7-8 minutes.
- Garnish with the coriander leaves. Serve hot.

French Beans Upkari

(French Beans with Coconut)

Serves 4

Ingredients

1 tbsp refined vegetable oil

½ tsp mustard seeds

½ tsp urad dhal*

2-3 red chillies, broken

500g/1lb 2oz French beans, chopped

1 tsp jaggery*, grated

Salt to taste

25g/scant 1oz fresh coconut, grated

Method

- Heat the oil in a saucepan. Add the mustard seeds. Let them splutter for 15 seconds.
- Add the dhal. Fry till golden brown. Add the remaining ingredients, except the coconut. Mix well. Cook on a low heat for 8-10 minutes.
- Garnish with the coconut. Serve hot.

Karatey Ambadey

(Bitter Gourd and Unripe Mango Curry)

Serves 4

Ingredients

250g/9oz bitter gourd*, sliced

Salt to taste

60g/2oz jaggery*, grated

1 tsp refined vegetable oil

4 dry red chillies

1 tsp urad dhal*

1 tsp fenugreek seeds

2 tsp coriander seeds

50g/1¾oz fresh coconut, grated

¼ tsp turmeric

4 small unripe mangoes

Method

- Rub the bitter gourd pieces with the salt. Set aside for an hour.

- Squeeze out the water from the gourd pieces. Cook them in a saucepan with the jaggery on a medium heat for 4-5 minutes. Set aside.

- Heat the oil in a saucepan. Add the red chillies, dhal, fenugreek and coriander seeds. Fry for a minute. Add the bitter gourd and the remaining ingredients. Mix well. Cook on a low heat for 4-5 minutes. Serve hot.

Kadhai Paneer

(Spicy Paneer)

Serves 4

Ingredients

2 tbsp refined vegetable oil

1 large onion, sliced

3 large green peppers, finely chopped

500g/1lb 2oz paneer*, chopped into 2.5cm/1in pieces

1 tomato, finely chopped

¼ tsp ground coriander, dry roasted (see cooking techniques)

Salt to taste

10g/¼oz coriander leaves, chopped

Method

- Heat the oil in a saucepan. Add the onion and peppers. Fry on a medium heat for 2-3 minutes.
- Add the remaining ingredients, except the coriander leaves. Mix well. Cook on a low heat for 5 minutes. Garnish with the coriander leaves. Serve hot.

Kathirikkai Vangi

(South Indian Aubergine Curry)

Serves 4

Ingredients

150g/5½oz masoor dhal*

Salt to taste

¼ tsp turmeric

500ml/16fl oz water

250g/9oz thin aubergines, sliced

1 tsp refined vegetable oil

¼ tsp mustard seeds

1 tsp tamarind paste

8-10 curry leaves

1 tsp sambhar powder*

Method

- Mix the masoor dhal with salt, a pinch of turmeric and half the water. Cook in a saucepan on a medium heat for 40 minutes. Set aside.

- Cook the aubergines with salt and the remaining turmeric and water in another saucepan on a medium heat for 20 minutes. Set aside.

- Heat the oil in a saucepan. Add the mustard seeds. Let them splutter for 15 seconds. Add the remaining ingredients, the dhal and the aubergine. Mix well. Simmer for 6-7 minutes. Serve hot.

Pitla

(Spicy Gram Flour Curry)

Serves 4

Ingredients

250g/9oz besan*

500ml/16fl oz water

2 tbsp refined vegetable oil

¼ tsp mustard seeds

2 large onions, finely chopped

6 garlic cloves, crushed

2 tbsp tamarind paste

1 tsp garam masala

Salt to taste

1 tbsp coriander leaves, chopped

Method

- Mix the besan and the water. Set aside.
- Heat the oil in a saucepan. Add the mustard seeds. Let them splutter for 15 seconds. Add the onions and garlic. Fry till the onions are brown.
- Add the besan paste. Cook on a low heat till it starts to boil.
- Add the remaining ingredients. Simmer for 5 minutes. Serve hot.

Cauliflower Masala

Serves 4

Ingredients

1 large cauliflower, parboiled (see cooking techniques) in salted water

3 tbsp refined vegetable oil

2 tbsp coriander leaves, finely chopped

1 tsp ground coriander

½ tsp ground cumin

¼ tsp ground ginger

Salt to taste

120ml/4fl oz water

For the sauce:

200g/7oz yoghurt

1 tbsp besan*, dry roasted (see cooking techniques)

¾ tsp chilli powder

Method

- Drain the cauliflower and chop into florets.
- Heat 2 tbsp oil in a frying pan. Add the cauliflower and fry it on a medium heat till golden brown. Set aside.
- Mix all the sauce ingredients together.
- Heat 1 tbsp oil in a saucepan and add this mixture. Fry for a minute.
- Cover with a lid and simmer for 8-10 minutes.
- Add the cauliflower. Mix well. Simmer for 5 minutes.
- Garnish with the coriander leaves. Serve hot.

Shukna Kacha Pepe

(Green Papaya Curry)

Serves 4

Ingredients

150g/5½oz chana dhal*, soaked overnight, drained and ground to a paste

3 tbsp refined vegetable oil plus for deep frying

2 whole dry red chillies

½ tsp fenugreek seeds

½ tsp mustard seeds

1 unripe papaya, peeled and grated

1 tsp turmeric

1 tbsp sugar

Salt to taste

Method

- Divide the dhal paste into walnut-sized balls. Flatten into thin discs.

- Heat the oil for deep frying in a frying pan. Add the discs. Deep fry on a medium heat till golden brown. Drain and break into small pieces. Set aside.

- Heat the remaining oil in a saucepan. Add the chillies, fenugreek and mustard seeds. Let them splutter for 15 seconds.

- Add the remaining ingredients. Mix well. Cover with a lid and cook on a low heat for 8-10 minutes. Add the dhal pieces. Mix well and serve.

Dry Okra

Ingredients

3 tbsp mustard oil

½ tsp kalonji seeds*

750g/1lb 10oz okra, slit lengthways

Salt to taste

½ tsp chilli powder

½ tsp turmeric

2 tsp sugar

3 tsp ground mustard

1 tbsp tamarind paste

Method

- Heat the oil in a saucepan. Fry the onion seeds and okra for 5 minutes.
- Add the salt, chilli powder, turmeric and sugar. Cover with a lid. Cook on a low heat for 10 minutes.
- Add the remaining ingredients. Mix well. Cook for 2-3 minutes. Serve hot.

Moghlai Cauliflower

Ingredients

5cm/2in root ginger

2 tsp cumin seeds

6-7 black peppercorns

500g/1lb 2oz cauliflower florets

Salt to taste

2 tbsp ghee

2 bay leaves

200g/7oz yoghurt

500ml/16fl oz coconut milk

1 tsp sugar

Method

- Grind the ginger, cumin seeds and peppercorns to a fine paste.
- Marinate the cauliflower florets with this paste and salt for 20 minutes.
- Heat the ghee in a frying pan. Add the florets. Fry till golden brown. Add the remaining ingredients. Mix well. Cover with a lid and simmer for 7-8 minutes. Serve hot.

Bhapa Shorshe Baingan

(Aubergine in Mustard Sauce)

Serves 4

Ingredients

2 long aubergines

Salt to taste

¼ tsp turmeric

3 tbsp refined vegetable oil

3 tbsp mustard oil

2–3 tbsp ready-made mustard

1 tbsp coriander leaves, finely chopped

1-2 green chillies, finely chopped

Method

- Slice each aubergine lengthways into 8-12 pieces. Marinate with the salt and turmeric for 5 minutes.

- Heat the oil in a saucepan. Add the aubergine slices and cover with a lid. Cook on a medium heat for 3-4 minutes, turning occasionally.

- Whisk the mustard oil with the ready-made mustard and add to the aubergines. Mix well. Cook on a medium heat for a minute.

- Garnish with the coriander leaves and green chillies. Serve hot.

Baked Vegetables in Spicy Sauce

Serves 4

Ingredients

2 tbsp butter

4 garlic cloves, finely chopped

1 large onion, finely chopped

1 tbsp plain white flour

200g/7oz frozen mixed vegetables

Salt to taste

1 tsp chilli powder

1 tsp mustard paste

250ml/8fl oz ketchup

4 large potatoes, boiled and sliced

250ml/8fl oz white sauce

4 tbsp grated Cheddar cheese

Method

- Heat the butter in a saucepan. Add the garlic and onion. Fry till translucent. Add the flour and fry for a minute.

- Add the vegetables, salt, chilli powder, mustard paste and ketchup. Cook on a medium heat for 4-5 minutes. Set aside.

- Grease a baking dish. Arrange the vegetable mixture and the potatoes in alternate layers. Pour the white sauce and cheese on top.

- Bake in an oven at 200°C (400°F, Gas Mark 6) for 20 minutes. Serve hot.

Tasty Tofu

Serves 4

Ingredients

2 tbsp refined vegetable oil

3 small onions, grated

1 tsp ginger paste

1 tsp garlic paste

3 tomatoes, puréed

50g/1¾oz Greek yoghurt, whisked

400g/14oz tofu, chopped into 2.5cm/1in pieces

25g/scant 1oz coriander leaves, finely chopped

Salt to taste

Method

- Heat the oil in a saucepan. Add the onions, ginger paste and garlic paste. Stir-fry for 5 minutes on a medium heat.
- Add the remaining ingredients. Mix well. Simmer for 3-4 minutes. Serve hot.

Aloo Baingan

(Potato and Aubergine Curry)

Serves 4

Ingredients

3 tbsp refined vegetable oil

1 tsp mustard seeds

½ tsp asafoetida

1cm/½in root ginger, finely chopped

4 green chillies, slit lengthways

10 garlic cloves, finely chopped

6 curry leaves

½ tsp turmeric

3 large potatoes, boiled and diced

250g/9oz aubergines, chopped

½ tsp amchoor*

Salt to taste

Method

- Heat the oil in a saucepan. Add the mustard seeds and asafoetida. Let them splutter for 15 seconds.

- Add the ginger, green chillies, garlic and curry leaves. Fry for 1 minute, stirring continuously.

- Add the remaining ingredients. Mix well. Cover with a lid and simmer for 10-12 minutes. Serve hot.

Sugar Snap Pea Curry

Serves 4

Ingredients

500g/1lb 2oz sugar snap peas

2 tbsp refined vegetable oil

1 tsp ginger paste

1 large onion, finely chopped

2 large potatoes, peeled and diced

½ tsp turmeric

½ tsp garam masala

½ tsp chilli powder

1 tsp sugar

2 large tomatoes, diced

Salt to taste

Method

- Peel the strings from the edges of the pea pods. Chop the pods. Set aside.
- Heat the oil in a saucepan. Add the ginger paste and onion. Fry till translucent. Add the remaining ingredients and the pods. Mix well. Cover with a lid and cook on a low heat for 7-8 minutes. Serve hot.

Potato Pumpkin Curry

Serves 4

Ingredients

2 tbsp refined vegetable oil

1 tsp panch phoron*

Pinch of asafoetida

1 dried red chilli, broken into bits

1 bay leaf

4 large potatoes, diced

200g/7oz pumpkin, diced

½ tsp ginger paste

½ tsp garlic paste

1 tsp ground cumin

1 tsp ground coriander

¼ tsp turmeric

½ tsp garam masala

1 tsp amchoor*

500ml/16fl oz water

Salt to taste

Method

- Heat the oil in a saucepan. Add the panch phoron. Let them splutter for 15 seconds.
- Add the asafoetida, red chilli pieces and the bay leaf. Fry for a minute.
- Add the remaining ingredients. Mix well. Simmer for 10-12 minutes. Serve hot.

Egg Thoran

(Spicy Scrambled Egg)

Serves 4

Ingredients

60ml/2fl oz refined vegetable oil

¼ tsp mustard seeds

2 onions, finely chopped

1 large tomato, finely chopped

1 tsp freshly ground black pepper

Salt to taste

4 eggs, whisked

25g/scant 1oz fresh coconut, grated

50g/1¾oz coriander leaves, chopped

Method

- Heat the oil in a saucepan and fry the mustard seeds. Let them splutter for 15 seconds. Add the onions and fry till brown. Add the tomato, pepper and salt. Fry for 2-3 minutes.
- Add the eggs. Cook on a low heat, scrambling continuously.
- Garnish with the coconut and coriander leaves. Serve hot.

Baingan Lajawab

(Aubergine with Cauliflower)

Serves 4

Ingredients

4 large aubergines

2 tbsp refined vegetable oil plus extra for deep frying

1 tsp cumin seeds

½ tsp turmeric

2.5cm/1in root ginger, ground

2 green chillies, finely chopped

1 tsp amchoor*

Salt to taste

100g/3½oz frozen peas

Method

- Slit each aubergine lengthways and scoop out the flesh.
- Heat the oil. Add the aubergine shells. Deep fry for 2 minutes. Set aside.
- Heat 2 tbsp oil in a saucepan. Add the cumin seeds and turmeric. Let them splutter for 15 seconds. Add the remaining ingredients and the aubergine flesh. Mash lightly and cook on a low heat for 5 minutes.
- Carefully stuff the aubergine shells with this mixture. Grill for 3-4 minutes. Serve hot.

Veggie Bahar

(Vegetables in a Nutty Sauce)

Serves 4

Ingredients

3 tbsp refined vegetable oil

1 large onion, finely chopped

2 large tomatoes, finely chopped

1 tsp ginger paste

1 tsp garlic paste

20 cashew nuts, ground

2 tbsp walnuts, ground

2 tbsp poppy seeds

200g/7oz yoghurt

100g/3½oz frozen mixed vegetables

1 tsp garam masala

Salt to taste

Method

- Heat the oil in a saucepan. Add the onion. Fry on a medium heat till brown. Add the tomatoes, ginger paste, garlic paste, cashew nuts, walnuts and poppy seeds. Fry for 3-4 minutes.

- Add the remaining ingredients. Cook for 7-8 minutes. Serve hot.

Stuffed Vegetables

Serves 4

Ingredients

4 small potatoes

100g/3½oz okra

4 small aubergines

4 tbsp refined vegetable oil

½ tsp mustard seeds

Pinch of asafoetida

For the filling:

250g/9oz besan*

1 tsp ground coriander

1 tsp ground cumin

½ tsp turmeric

1 tsp chilli powder

1 tsp garam masala

Salt to taste

Method

- Mix all the filling ingredients together. Set aside.
- Slit the potatoes, okra and aubergines. Stuff with the filling. Set aside.
- Heat the oil in a saucepan. Add the mustard seeds and asafoetida. Let them splutter for 15 seconds. Add the stuffed vegetables. Cover with a lid and cook on a low heat for 8-10 minutes. Serve hot.

Singhi Aloo

(Drumsticks with Potatoes)

Serves 4

Ingredients

5 tbsp refined vegetable oil

3 small onions, finely chopped

3 green chillies, finely chopped

2 large tomatoes, finely chopped

2 tsp ground coriander

Salt to taste

5 Indian drumsticks*, chopped into 7.5cm/3in pieces

2 large potatoes, chopped

360ml/12fl oz water

Method

- Heat the oil in a saucepan. Add the onions and chillies. Fry them on a low heat for a minute.

- Add the tomatoes, ground coriander and salt. Fry for 2-3 minutes.

- Add the drumsticks, potatoes and water. Mix well. Simmer for 10-12 minutes. Serve hot.

Sindhi Curry

Serves 4

Ingredients

150g/5½oz masoor dhal*

Salt to taste

1 litre/1¾ pints water

4 tomatoes, finely chopped

5 tbsp refined vegetable oil

½ tsp cumin seeds

¼ tsp fenugreek seeds

8 curry leaves

3 green chillies, slit lengthways

¼ tsp asafoetida

4 tbsp besan*

½ tsp chilli powder

½ tsp turmeric

8 okras, slit lengthways

10 French beans, diced

6-7 kokum*

1 large carrot, julienned

1 large potato, diced

Method

- Mix the dhal with the salt and water. Cook this mixture in a saucepan on a medium heat for 45 minutes, stirring occasionally.
- Add the tomatoes and simmer for 7-8 minutes. Set aside.
- Heat the oil in a saucepan. Add the cumin and fenugreek seeds, curry leaves, green chillies and asafoetida. Let them splutter for 30 seconds.
- Add the besan. Fry for a minute, stirring constantly.
- Add the remaining ingredients and the dhal mixture. Mix thoroughly. Simmer for 10 minutes. Serve hot.

Dum Gobhi

(Slow Cooked Cauliflower)

Serves 4

Ingredients

2.5cm/1in root ginger, julienned

2 tomatoes, finely chopped

¼ tsp turmeric

1 tbsp yoghurt

½ tsp garam masala

Salt to taste

800g/1¾lb cauliflower florets

Method

- Mix together all the ingredients, except the cauliflower florets.
- Place the cauliflower florets in a saucepan and pour this mixture over it. Cover with a lid and simmer for 20 minutes, stirring occasionally. Serve hot.

Chhole

(Chickpea Curry)

Serves 5

Ingredients

375g/13oz chickpeas, soaked overnight

1 litre/1¾ pints water

Salt to taste

1 tomato, finely chopped

3 small onions, finely chopped

1½ tbsp coriander leaves, finely chopped

2 tbsp refined vegetable oil

1 tsp cumin seeds

1 tsp ginger paste

1 tsp garlic paste

2 bay leaves

1 tsp sugar

1 tsp chilli powder

½ tsp turmeric

1 tbsp ghee

4 green chillies, slit lengthways

½ tsp ground cinnamon

½ tsp ground clove

Juice of 1 lemon

Method

- Mix the chickpeas with half the water and the salt. Cook this mixture in a saucepan on a medium heat for 30 minutes. Remove from the heat and drain the chickpeas.
- Grind 2 tbsp of the chickpeas with half of the tomato, one onion and half the coriander leaves to a fine paste. Set aside.
- Heat the oil in a large saucepan. Add the cumin seeds. Let them splutter for 15 seconds.
- Add the remaining onions, the ginger paste and the garlic paste. Fry this mixture on a medium heat till the onions are brown.
- Add the remaining tomato along with the bay leaves, sugar, chilli powder, turmeric and the chickpea-tomato paste. Fry this mixture on a medium heat for 2-3 minutes.
- Add the remaining chickpeas with the remaining water. Simmer for 8-10 minutes. Set aside.
- Heat the ghee in a small saucepan. Add the green chillies, ground cinnamon and clove. Let them splutter for 30 seconds. Pour this mixture over the chickpeas. Mix well. Sprinkle the lemon juice and the remaining coriander leaves on top of the chhole. Serve hot.

Aubergine Curry with Onion & Potato

Serves 4

Ingredients

3 tbsp refined vegetable oil

2 large onions, finely chopped

1 tsp ginger paste

1 tsp garlic paste

1 tsp ground coriander

1 tsp ground cumin

1 tsp chilli powder

¼ tsp turmeric

120ml/4fl oz water

Salt to taste

250g/9oz small aubergines

250g/9oz baby potatoes, halved

50g/1¾oz coriander leaves, finely chopped

Method

- Heat the oil in a saucepan. Add the onions. Fry till they turn translucent.
- Add the remaining ingredients, except the coriander leaves. Mix well. Simmer for 15 minutes.
- Garnish with the coriander leaves. Serve hot.

Simple Bottle Gourd

Serves 4

Ingredients

½ tbsp ghee

1 tsp cumin seeds

2 green chillies, slit lengthways

750g/1lb 10oz bottle gourd*, chopped

Salt to taste

120ml/4fl oz milk

1 tbsp desiccated coconut

10g/¼oz coriander leaves, finely chopped

Method

- Heat the ghee in a saucepan. Add the cumin seeds and green chillies. Let them splutter for 15 seconds.
- Add the bottle gourd, salt and milk. Simmer for 10-12 minutes.
- Add the remaining ingredients. Mix well. Serve hot.

Mixed Vegetable Curry

Serves 4

Ingredients

3 tbsp refined vegetable oil

1 tsp cumin seeds

1 tsp ground coriander

½ tsp ground cumin

1 tsp chilli powder

¼ tsp turmeric

½ tsp sugar

1 carrot, chopped into strips

1 large potato, diced

200g/7oz French beans, chopped

50g/1¾oz cauliflower florets

Salt to taste

200g/7oz tomato purée

120ml/4fl oz water

10g/¼oz coriander leaves, finely chopped

Method

- Heat the oil in a saucepan. Add the cumin seeds, ground coriander and ground cumin. Let them splutter for 15 seconds.
- Add the remaining ingredients, except the coriander leaves. Mix thoroughly. Simmer for 15 minutes.
- Garnish the curry with the coriander leaves. Serve hot.

Dry Mixed Vegetables

Serves 4

Ingredients

3 tbsp refined vegetable oil

1 tsp cumin seeds

1 tsp ground coriander

½ tsp ground cumin

¼ tsp turmeric

1 carrot, julienned

1 large potato, diced

200g/7oz French beans, chopped

60g/2oz cauliflower florets

Salt to taste

120ml/4fl oz water

10g/¼oz coriander leaves, chopped

Method

- Heat the oil in a saucepan. Add the cumin seeds. Let them splutter for 15 seconds.

- Add the remaining ingredients, except the coriander leaves. Mix thoroughly and cook for 15 minutes on a low heat.

- Garnish with the coriander leaves and serve hot.

Dry Potatoes & Peas

Serves 4

Ingredients

3 tbsp refined vegetable oil

1 tsp cumin seeds

½ tsp turmeric

1 tsp garam masala

2 large potatoes, boiled and diced

400g/14oz cooked peas

Salt to taste

Method

- Heat the oil in a saucepan. Add the cumin seeds and turmeric. Let them splutter for 15 seconds.
- Add the remaining ingredients. Stir-fry on a medium heat for 5 minutes. Serve hot.

Dhokar Dhalna

(Bengal Gram Curry)

Serves 4

Ingredients

300g/10oz chana dhal*, soaked overnight

2 tbsp mustard oil

1 tsp cumin seeds

Salt to taste

5cm/2in cinnamon

4 green cardamom pods

6 cloves

½ tsp turmeric

½ tsp sugar

250ml/8fl oz water

3 large potatoes, diced and fried

Method

- Grind the chana dhal with enough water to form a smooth paste. Set aside.

- Heat half the oil in a saucepan. Add half the cumin seeds. Let them splutter for 15 seconds. Add the dhal paste and the salt. Fry for 2-3 minutes. Drain and spread on a large plate and allow to set. Chop into 2.5cm/1in pieces. Set aside.

- Fry these dhal pieces in the remaining oil till golden brown. Set aside.

- In the same oil, add the remaining ingredients, except the potatoes. Cook for 2 minutes. Add the potatoes and the dhal pieces. Mix well. Cook on a low heat for 4-5 minutes. Serve hot.

Spicy Fried Potatoes

Serves 4

Ingredients

250ml/8fl oz refined vegetable oil

3 large potatoes, chopped into thin strips

½ tsp chilli powder

1 tsp freshly ground black pepper

Salt to taste

Method

- Heat the oil in a saucepan. Add the potato strips. Deep fry them on a medium heat till they turn golden brown.
- Drain and toss well with the remaining ingredients. Serve hot.

CPSIA information can be obtained
at www.ICGtesting.com
Printed in the USA
BVHW080229190521
607644BV00013B/1234

9 781801 989220